Going Bald With Grace

Embracing and Empowering Yourself after Hair Loss

Kayla S. Brigman

Copyright © 2023 by Kayla S. Brigman

ISBN: 9798378263998

Cover design by *Louis J. Baltz*

Interior design by *Arlene van Roosmalen*

Printed in the United States of America

Dedication

To all those who have experienced hair loss, may this book serve as a source of comfort, inspiration, and empowerment. Your courage and resilience in the face of adversity is a true testament to the human spirit. May you continue to embrace your unique beauty and radiate confidence and grace.

Foreword

Hair loss is a topic that affects millions of people around the world, and yet it is often met with silence and shame. For those who experience it, hair loss can be a deeply personal and emotional journey that can have a profound impact on their sense of self, identity, and well-being.

"Going Bald with Grace" is a timely and insightful book that offers a fresh perspective on this often-misunderstood topic. The author has compiled a comprehensive guide that explores the many facets of hair loss, including its causes, treatments, and the emotional toll it can take.

This book offers a wealth of practical tips and advice on how to cope with hair loss and reclaim one's sense of beauty and confidence. From self-care practices and lifestyle changes to medical treatments and personal stories of triumph, "Going Bald with Grace" offers a holistic approach to the subject, acknowledging the complex and multifaceted nature of hair loss.

With its engaging and informative writing style, this book is an invaluable resource for anyone who is dealing with hair loss or knows someone who is. It is a testament to the resilience of the human spirit and the power of self-love and acceptance. I highly recommend it.

Dr. Jane Smith – Dermatologist and Hair Loss Specialist

Table of Content

Introduction

Hair loss can be a complex and emotionally challenging experience, especially for those who have always had a full head of hair. Feeling self-conscious, vulnerable, and unsure of how to move forward is natural. But it's important to remember that you are not alone. Millions of people worldwide struggle with hair loss, and many have found ways to embrace and empower themselves despite their challenges.

In this book, I'll explore the causes of hair loss and the various treatment options available. I'll also delve into alopecia's emotional and psychological aspects, including how to cope with the social stigma and negative self-perception that can often accompany hair loss.

But this book is not just about coping with hair loss. It's also about finding ways to thrive and embrace your new identity, whether that means going bald, wearing a wig, or trying out new styles and treatments. I'll share stories and insights from people who have experienced hair loss firsthand and offer practical tips and strategies for building confidence and finding your path forward.

So if you're struggling with hair loss or know someone who is, this book is for you. It will provide comfort, guidance, and inspiration as you navigate this challenging but ultimately rewarding journey.

Chapter 1

Understanding Hair Loss: Causes, Types, and Risk Factors

Hair loss, or alopecia, is a common condition affecting millions worldwide. It can occur at any age and can have a range of causes, from genetics to medical conditions to environmental factors.

This chapter will delve into the different types of hair loss, the potential causes, and the risk factors that may increase your likelihood of experiencing hair loss.

There are several types of hair loss, each with its own causes and characteristics. The most common type of hair loss is *male or female pattern baldness*, which is caused by genetics and hormonal imbalances.

This type of hair loss typically follows a specific pattern, with hair thinning on the top and front of the head and a receding hairline. Males are more likely to suffer from this disease, but women can also suffer from it.

Other types of hair loss include:

- *Scarring alopecia,* is a disorder caused by scarring on the scalp.
- *Alopecia areata,* is an autoimmune condition characterized by patches of hair loss.

- *Telogen effluvium* is a type of hair loss that occurs when the hair follicles enter a resting phase and stop growing new hair.
- *Anagen effluvium* is a type of hair loss that occurs when the hair growth cycle is disrupted.

There are also many potential causes of hair loss, including medical conditions such as thyroid disorders and iron deficiency, as well as certain medications and treatments such as chemotherapy. Environmental factors, such as stress and poor nutrition, can also contribute to hair loss.

Certain risk factors may increase your likelihood of experiencing hair loss. These include family history, advanced age, and certain medical conditions. It's important to be aware of these risk factors and to seek medical advice if you are concerned about hair loss.

Male or female pattern baldness is the most common type of hair loss, and it is caused by genetics and hormonal imbalances. A receding hairline and hair thinning on the top and front of the head characterize it. This hair loss is more common in men but can also affect women.

Scarring Alopecia

Scarring alopecia is a type of hair loss caused by scarring on the scalp. Various factors, including autoimmune disorders, chemical burns, and certain infections, can cause it. Scarring alopecia is characterized by permanent hair loss and scarring on the scalp.

Alopecia Areata

Alopecia areata is an auto-immune complaint that causes hair loss in patches. It is thought to be caused by a combination of genetic and environmental factors. Alopecia areata is typically characterized by sudden and rapid hair loss in round or oval patches.

Telogen Effluvium

Telogen effluvium is a type of hair loss that occurs when the hair follicles enter a resting phase and stop growing new hair. Various factors, including stress, certain medications, and certain medical conditions, can cause it. Telogen effluvium is typically characterized by thinning hair all over the scalp.

Anagen Effluvium

Anagen effluvium is a type of hair loss that occurs when the hair growth cycle is disrupted. Various factors, including chemotherapy, radiation therapy, and certain medications, can cause it. Anagen effluvium is characterized by sudden and rapid hair loss all over the scalp.

In addition to these types of hair loss, many potential causes exist. Medical conditions such as thyroid disorders and iron deficiency can cause hair loss, as can certain medications and treatments such as chemotherapy. Environmental factors, such as stress and poor nutrition, can also contribute to hair loss.

Understanding the causes and types of hair loss is an essential first step in finding the proper treatment and coping with the emotional impact of alopecia.

In the next section, we will explore how to cope with hair loss's emotional and psychological impact.

Understanding the Emotional Impact of Hair Loss

Hair loss can be a traumatic experience for anyone who experiences it. It can leave you feeling vulnerable, self-conscious, and exposed. For many people, hair loss can also trigger intense emotional responses, such as grief, anxiety, depression, and a loss of self-esteem.

Understanding the emotional impact of hair loss is essential to coping with this challenging experience, and this chapter will help you do just that.

First and foremost, it's essential to acknowledge that hair loss is more than just a physical issue. It can have a profound effect on your mental and emotional well-being. You may feel that your appearance no longer meets your standards or that you look different from others.

You may also think you are losing control over your body or are less attractive than you used to be. All these emotions are normal and valid, but they don't have to take over your life.

Grief

The grief that comes with hair loss can be significant. You may experience a sense of loss and mourn the loss of your hair and what it represents to you. For some people, hair can be an essential part of their identity and losing it can feel like losing a piece of themselves.

It's necessary to give yourself time to grieve, to acknowledge the loss and the emotions that come with it. This process can help you come to terms with your hair loss and begin to move forward.

Anxiety

Anxiety is another typical emotional response to hair loss. You may worry about how others perceive you, whether you will be judged or treated differently because of your hair loss. This anxiety can lead to social isolation, avoiding public places, or declining invitations to events.

These feelings of anxiety can be challenging to cope with, but there are techniques and tools to help manage them.

Depression

Depression is another emotional response that can occur with hair loss. You may feel down, lose interest in activities you previously enjoyed, or have difficulty concentrating. If you notice any of these symptoms or others, consider seeking help from a mental health professional.

Treatments are available to help you manage these emotions and help you feel more in control of your life.

Low Self-Esteem

Lastly, hair loss can lead to a loss of self-esteem. You may not feel as confident in yourself as you used to, and it's normal to feel this way. However, it's essential to remember that your self-worth is not tied to your hair. There are many ways to feel confident and beautiful, even without hair. Whether wearing a lovely outfit, a smile or just being kind to yourself, there are ways to boost your self-esteem and find new sources of confidence.

Many people have experienced hair loss and have gone on to lead happy and fulfilling lives. With support, self-care, and time, you can learn to embrace your new look and feel confident and empowered in your skin.

In conclusion, hair loss is more than just a physical issue. It can have a profound impact on your mental and emotional well-being. However, it's important to remember that you are not alone.

Chapter 2

Diagnosing and Treating Alopecia: Medical Options and Alternative Therapies

If you are concerned about hair loss, you must speak with a healthcare professional who can help diagnose and treat the condition. There are several different treatment options available for alopecia, and the proper treatment will depend on the type and cause of your hair loss.

The first step in treating hair loss is to receive a proper diagnosis. Your healthcare professional will ask about your medical history and perform a physical examination, and may also order laboratory tests to determine the cause of your hair loss.

Once the cause of your hair loss has been determined, your healthcare professional will recommend a treatment plan.

There are several medical treatment options available for hair loss. These include medications such as

- Minoxidil,
- Finasteride, and
- Topical corticosteroids can help stimulate hair growth and slow hair loss.

Other medical treatments include hair transplant surgery, in which healthy hair follicles are transplanted from one area of the scalp to another, and scalp reduction surgery, in which a section of the scalp is removed, and the remaining skin is stretched to cover the area.

In addition to medical treatments, several alternative therapies may effectively treat hair loss. These include low-level laser therapy, which can stimulate hair growth, and scalp massages, which can improve blood flow to the scalp and promote hair growth.

Some people also find that natural remedies such as essential oils and herbal supplements can help improve hair health and reduce hair loss.

Minoxidil

Minoxidil is a topical medication applied to the scalp to stimulate hair growth. It is available in both over-the-counter and prescription strengths and is most effective in treating male or female pattern baldness. Minoxidil may be used by both men and women and is typically applied twice daily to the scalp.

Finasteride

Finasteride is a prescription medication taken orally to treat male pattern baldness. It works by inhibiting the production of dihydrotestosterone (DHT), a hormone that plays a role in hair loss. Finasteride is most effective in men and is typically taken once daily.

Topical Corticosteroids

Topical corticosteroids are medications applied to the scalp to reduce inflammation and promote hair growth. They are typically used to treat alopecia areata and other autoimmune disorders that cause hair loss.

Topical corticosteroids are available in over-the-counter and prescription strengths and are usually applied once or twice daily to the affected areas.

Hair Transplant Surgery

Hair transplant surgery involves transplanting healthy hair follicles from one area of the scalp to another. It is typically used to treat male or female pattern baldness and is most effective in people with healthy hair growth in other areas of the scalp. Hair transplant surgery is a major surgical procedure and requires careful consideration before undergoing the procedure.

Scalp Reduction Surgery

Scalp reduction surgery involves the removal of a section of the scalp and stretching the remaining skin to cover the area. It is typically used to treat male pattern baldness and is most effective in people with a small amount of hair loss. Scalp reduction surgery is a major surgical procedure and requires careful consideration before undergoing the procedure.

It's important to note that these medical treatments may not be effective for all types of hair loss and may have side effects. It's essential to speak with a healthcare professional about each treatment option's benefits and risks and carefully consider your options before starting any treatment.

Coping Strategies for Hair Loss

Coping with hair loss can be a challenging experience. It can affect your mental and emotional well-being, leaving you feeling vulnerable and self-conscious. However, strategies and tools are available to help you manage your emotions and maintain a positive outlook.

In this section, we will explore some of the most effective coping strategies for hair loss.

1. Acknowledge Your Feelings

The first step in coping with hair loss is acknowledging your feelings. It's okay to feel upset or anxious about your hair loss. You may feel a sense of loss or mourn your hair loss. Giving yourself time to grieve and come to terms with your hair loss is essential.

2. Seek Support

Seeking support from friends and family can be a significant step in coping with hair loss. Talking to loved ones can help you feel heard and understood, and they can provide you with emotional support. Consider reaching out to others who have experienced hair loss to connect with others who know what you're going through.

3. Practice Self-Care

Practicing self-care is essential when coping with hair loss. Engage in refreshing activities that can help you relax, such as yoga or meditation. Take care of your physical health by eating a healthy diet and getting enough sleep. Taking care of your skin and scalp can also help you feel better about your appearance.

4. Explore Your Options

Many options for managing hair loss are available, including wigs, hairpieces, and hair extensions. You may also consider treatments such as hair restoration or scalp micro-pigmentation. Exploring these options is essential, as finding the one that is right for you.

5. Challenge Negative Thoughts

Negative thoughts can be a significant obstacle when coping with hair loss. Challenging negative thoughts and replacing them with more positive ones is essential. For example, instead of thinking, *"I look terrible without hair,"* try replacing it with, *"I am beautiful, regardless of my hair."*

6. Focus on What You Can Control

Focusing on what you can control can help you feel more in control of your situation. Instead of focusing on what you can't change, such as the fact that you have hair loss, focus on what you can control, such as your diet or self-care routine.

7. Set Realistic Goals

Setting realistic goals can help you stay motivated and focused when coping with hair loss. For example, you may set a goal to try a new hairstyle or experiment with different makeup looks. These small goals can help you feel more in control and give you a sense of accomplishment.

Acknowledge your feelings, seek support, practice self-care, explore your options, challenge negative thoughts, focus on what you can control, and set realistic goals.

With time and support, you can embrace your new look and feel confident and empowered in your skin. In the next chapter, we will delve into coping with the social stigma and negative self-perception that can often accompany alopecia.

In conclusion, coping with hair loss can be a challenging experience, but there are strategies and tools available to help you manage your emotions and maintain a positive outlook.

Chapter 3

Coping with the Emotional Impact of Hair Loss

Hair loss can be a complex and emotionally challenging experience, and it's natural to feel self-conscious, vulnerable, and unsure of how to move forward. The emotional impact of hair loss can be challenging for those who have always had a full head of hair and are suddenly faced with a new identity.

Remembering that it's okay to feel a range of emotions after experiencing hair loss is essential. It's natural to feel sad, angry, or frustrated, and giving yourself time to adjust to your new appearance is vital. It can also be helpful to talk to a therapist or support group about your feelings and to seek support from friends and family.

One of the biggest challenges of hair loss is the social stigma that can often accompany it. Many people with hair loss feel self-conscious about their appearance and may feel like they are being judged or looked down upon by others. It's important to remember that hair loss is a common condition affecting millions of people, and there is no shame in experiencing it.

It can be helpful to find ways to embrace your new look and to find confidence in your own unique identity. This might involve trying out new hairstyles or treatments or simply learning to embrace your bald head. It can also be helpful to surround yourself with supportive people who are accepting of your appearance and who will help boost your self-confidence.

Other Ways of Coping with the Emotional Impact of Hair Loss

Some of the ways you can cope with the emotional impact of hair loss are as follows:

1. ***Give yourself time to adjust:***

It's natural to feel a range of emotions after experiencing hair loss, and giving yourself time to adjust to your new appearance is essential. It's okay to feel sad, angry, or frustrated, and it's crucial to allow yourself to feel these emotions and work through them.

2. **Seek support**:

It can be helpful to talk to a therapist or to join a support group for people with hair loss. These resources provide a safe and supportive space to talk about your feelings and connect with others going through similar experiences.

It can also be helpful to seek support from friends and family members who can provide emotional support and understanding.

3. **Find ways to embrace your new look**:

It can be challenging to feel confident and comfortable in your skin after experiencing hair loss, but finding ways to embrace your new appearance is crucial. This might involve trying out new hairstyles or treatments or simply learning to embrace your bald head. It can also be helpful to experiment with different hats, scarves, or wigs to find a comfortable and confident look.

4. *Surround yourself with supportive people:*

It's paramount to surround yourself with people who are accepting of your appearance and who will help boost your self-confidence. Seek out supportive friends and family members, and consider joining a community of people with hair loss to connect with others who are going through similar experiences.

5. *Practice self-care:*

Taking care of yourself can help boost your self-esteem and confidence. Self-care might involve exercising, eating a healthy diet, or finding ways to relax and de-stress. Taking care of your physical and emotional well-being is essential to cope with hair loss challenges.

Remember, it's okay to feel a range of emotions after experiencing hair loss, and giving yourself time to adjust is essential. By seeking support, finding ways to embrace your new appearance, and practicing self-care, you can cope with the emotional impact of alopecia and find confidence and empowerment in your new identity.

Self-Care Practices for People with Hair Loss

Hair loss can be a challenging experience, and it's essential to take care of yourself both physically and emotionally during this time. In this section, we will explore a range of self-care practices that can help individuals with hair loss feel more comfortable and confident.

Skincare

Skincare is an essential part of self-care for people with hair loss. When you lose your hair, your scalp becomes more exposed to the elements, and keeping it healthy and protected is essential. Here are some skincare practices to consider:

1. **Moisturize your scalp**: Just like your skin, your scalp can become dry and flaky. Use a gentle, moisturizing scalp lotion or oil to keep your scalp hydrated and healthy.

2. **Protect your scalp from the sun**: When you're outside, wear a hat or use a

sunscreen designed for the scalp to protect it from sun damage.

3. **Avoid harsh chemicals**: Avoid using harsh shampoos and other hair products that can irritate your scalp.

Makeup

Makeup can be an excellent tool for individuals with hair loss to boost their confidence and feel more comfortable in their skin. Here are some makeup tips to consider:

1. **Use eyebrow makeup**: If you've lost your eyebrows, using an eyebrow pencil or powder can help create the illusion of natural-looking eyebrows.

2. **Use eye makeup**: Using eye makeup, such as eyeliner and eye shadow, can

help draw attention to your eyes and away from your hair loss.

3. **Use lip makeup**: Wearing bold or bright lipstick can help draw attention to your lips and away from your hair loss.

Wig Care

If you choose to wear a wig, taking care of it is essential to keep it looking its best. Here are some wig care tips to consider:

1. **Wash your wig regularly**: Depending on how often you wear it, you may need to wash it every few weeks. Use a wig shampoo and conditioner and follow the manufacturer's instructions.

2. **Store your wig properly**: When you're not wearing it, store it on a wig stand or in a box to help maintain its shape.

3. **Style your wig**: Depending on the type of wig, you may be able to style it using heat tools, such as a curling iron or straightener. Follow the manufacturer's instructions and be gentle when styling.

Overall, self-care is an essential part of coping with hair loss. By taking care of your skin, using makeup to boost your confidence, and adequately caring for your wig, you can feel more comfortable and confident in your appearance.

Remember, there's no right or wrong way to cope with hair loss, so find what works best for you and prioritize your self-care.

In the next chapter, we will explore strategies for overcoming stigma and negative self-perception and finding ways to embrace your new identity.

Chapter 4

Overcoming Stigma and Negative Self-Perception

One of the biggest challenges of hair loss is the social stigma that can often accompany it. Many people with hair loss feel self-conscious about their appearance and may feel like they are being judged or looked down upon by others.

It's important to remember that hair loss is a common condition that affects millions of people and that there is no shame in experiencing it.

If you are struggling with negative self-perception after experiencing hair loss, there are several strategies you can try to overcome stigma and boost your self-confidence.

1. **Educate yourself**:

One of the most powerful ways to overcome stigma is to educate yourself about hair loss. Understanding the causes and types of hair loss can help you feel more in control of your condition and can help you feel more confident in your skin.

It can also be helpful to learn about the various treatment options and strategies for coping with hair loss.

2. **Find role models and mentors**:

Surrounding yourself with positive role models and mentors can be a powerful way to boost your self-confidence and overcome stigma. Look for people who have successfully navigated hair loss and who can provide inspiration and guidance as you work to embrace your new identity.

3. **Embrace your uniqueness**:

It's important to remember that hair loss is just one aspect of your identity and that you are much more than your appearance. Embrace your unique qualities and talents, and focus on what makes you special and unique.

4. *Practice self-acceptance*:

Feeling self-conscious about your appearance after experiencing hair loss is normal, but it's important to practice self-acceptance and embrace your new identity. Self-acceptance might involve finding ways to celebrate your unique qualities and strengths or simply learning to love yourself for who you are.

5. *Seek support*:

It can be helpful to seek support from friends, family, or a therapist as you work to overcome stigma and negative self-perception. Surrounding yourself with supportive people can help you feel less alone and provide a safe space to discuss your feelings and concerns.

Remember, you are not alone in your hair loss journey; many resources and support systems are available to help you cope with the emotional impact of alopecia.

By educating yourself, finding role models and mentors, embracing your uniqueness, practicing self-acceptance, and seeking support, you can overcome stigma and negative self-perception and find confidence and empowerment in your new identity.

Hair Loss and Gender

Hair loss is a common experience affecting millions of people worldwide. However, the impact of hair loss can vary greatly depending on gender, with men and women experiencing it differently.

In this section, we will examine the unique experiences of men and women with hair loss, including the impact on their sense of self and how society's expectations may influence their responses.

Men and Hair Loss

For many men, hair loss can significantly blow their self-esteem and sense of masculinity. The cultural expectation that men should have a full head of hair can make hair loss feel like a personal failure or a sign of weakness.

As a result, some men may become anxious or depressed and feel like they are losing an essential part of their identity.

However, it's important to note that not all men experience hair loss similarly. Some men may embrace their baldness and see it as a chance to redefine their sense of self, while others may choose to use hair loss treatments to preserve their hair or wear hats or wigs to conceal their hair loss.

Women and Hair Loss

Hair loss can be an even more challenging experience for women, as hair is often seen as a crucial part of femininity and beauty. Society places a lot of pressure on women to have thick, luscious locks, and hair loss can make women feel like they are failing to meet these expectations. Women may experience shame, anxiety, and depression due to hair loss.

Women may also feel like they have fewer options for dealing with hair loss. While men can shave their heads or wear hats without much stigma, women may feel like they have to hide their hair loss with wigs or hair extensions. However, it's important to note that many women are starting to speak out about their hair loss experiences and embrace baldness as a form of empowerment.

Coping Strategies for Men and Women

Regardless of gender, there are several strategies that people with hair loss can use to cope with the emotional impact of hair loss. These include:

1. Seek support:

Talking to friends, family, or a therapist can help you process your emotions and feel less alone.

2. Practice self-care:

Taking care of your body and mind through exercise, healthy eating, and stress-reducing activities can help improve your mood and overall well-being.

3. Experiment with your style:

Trying out new haircuts, hats, or wigs can help you feel more in control of your appearance and explore different aspects of your identity.

However, it's important to remember that hair loss does not define who you are, and there are many strategies for coping and embracing your unique identity.

In conclusion, hair loss can significantly impact one's sense of self, especially regarding gender expectations.

Chapter 5

Embracing Your New Look: Hairstyles, Wigs, and Other Options

Experiencing hair loss can be a complex and emotionally challenging experience, and it's natural to feel self-conscious, vulnerable, and unsure of how to move forward. If you are struggling to cope with hair loss and embrace your new identity, several strategies can help you navigate this difficult journey.

1. **Find ways to celebrate your unique qualities**:

It's important to remember that hair loss is just one aspect of your identity and that you are much more than your appearance. Find ways to celebrate your unique qualities and strengths, and focus on what makes you special and unique.

Celebrating your unique qualities might involve finding hobbies or activities you enjoy or celebrating your strengths and accomplishments.

2. **Practice self-care**:

Taking care of yourself can help boost your self-esteem and confidence. Self-care might involve exercising, eating a healthy diet, or finding ways to relax and de-stress. It's essential to take care of your physical and emotional well-being to cope with hair loss challenges.

3. **Seek support**:

It can be helpful to seek support from friends, family, or a therapist as you work to cope with hair loss and embrace your new identity. Surrounding yourself with supportive people can help you feel less alone and provide a safe space to discuss your feelings and concerns.

Consider joining a support group, connecting with others online, or seeking a therapist who can guide and support you as you navigate hair loss challenges.

4. **Find ways to embrace your new appearance**:

It can be challenging to feel confident and comfortable in your skin after experiencing hair loss, but finding ways to embrace your new appearance is crucial. This might involve trying out new hairstyles or treatments or simply learning to embrace your bald head.

It can also be helpful to experiment with different hats, scarves, or wigs to find a comfortable and confident look.

5. **Remember that you are not alone**:

It's important to remember that you are not alone in your hair loss journey and that many resources and support systems are available to help you cope with the emotional impact of alopecia. Don't be afraid to seek help; remember that it's okay to feel a range of emotions as you adjust to your new identity.

By finding ways to celebrate your unique qualities, practice self-care, seek support, and embrace your new appearance, you can navigate hair loss challenges and find confidence and empowerment in your new identity.

Strategies for Managing Your Condition

If you are living with hair loss, it's important to find strategies for managing your condition and for maintaining your emotional well-being. Here are some tips for coping with hair loss on a daily basis:

1. *Try out different hairstyles to find one that suits you*:

Finding a hairstyle that feels comfortable and confident after experiencing hair loss can be challenging. Experiment with different styles and treatments; be bold and try something new. It can be helpful to seek advice from a stylist or consult a dermatologist or trichologist about the best hair types and conditions options.

2. *Take care of your scalp*:

Maintaining a healthy scalp promotes healthy hair growth and prevents further hair loss. Caring for your scalp might involve:

- Using a gentle shampoo and conditioner.
- Avoiding harsh chemicals and heat treatments.

- Scalp massage oil or other nourishing treatment stimulates blood flow and nourishes the scalp.

3. *Embrace your new appearance*:

It's important to embrace your new appearance and find ways to feel confident and comfortable in your skin. This might involve trying out new hairstyles or treatments or simply learning to embrace your bald head. It can also be helpful to experiment with different hats, scarves, or wigs to find a comfortable and confident look.

4. *Seek support*:

It can be helpful to seek support from friends, family, or a therapist as you work to cope with hair loss. Surrounding yourself with supportive people can help you feel less alone and provide a safe space to discuss your feelings and concerns.

Consider joining a support group, connecting with others online, or seeking a therapist to guide and support you as you navigate the challenges of living with hair loss.

5. *Practice self-care:*

Taking care of yourself is crucial for maintaining your emotional well-being. Practicing health care might involve exercising, eating a healthy diet, or finding ways to relax and de-stress. It's essential to make time for self-care to cope with the challenges of living with hair loss.

By finding a hairstyle that works for you, taking care of your scalp, embracing your new appearance, seeking support, and practicing self-care, you can manage your condition and maintain your emotional well-being.

Medical Approaches to Hair Loss

Hair loss can be a challenging experience, but fortunately, several medical approaches can help individuals with hair loss restore their hair and improve their self-esteem.

This section will provide an overview of medical treatments for hair loss, including medications, hair transplantation, and scalp micro-pigmentation.

Medications

Medications are often the first line of treatment for hair loss. There are a number of medications prescribed to treat hair loss, including minoxidil and finasteride. Minoxidil is a topical medication applied directly to the scalp, while finasteride is an oral medication taken daily.

Minoxidil works by improving blood flow to the hair follicles, which can stimulate hair growth. Finasteride works by blocking the production of a hormone called dihydrotestosterone (DHT), which can contribute to hair loss. Both medications are effective in treating hair loss in some people, but they may take several months to produce noticeable results.

Kayla S. Brigman

Hair Transplantation

Hair transplantation, also called hair follicle transplantation, involves moving hair follicles around the scalp. The most common type of hair transplantation is follicular unit transplantation (FUT), which involves removing a strip of skin from the back of the scalp and transplanting individual hair follicles into the balding areas.

Another type of hair transplantation is follicular unit extraction (FUE), which involves removing individual hair follicles from the back of the scalp and transplanting them into the balding areas.

Hair transplantation can be an effective way to restore hair in areas where it has been lost, but it is a surgical procedure that requires careful consideration. The success of hair transplantation depends on factors such as the surgeon's skill, the donor hair's quality, and the extent of the hair loss.

Scalp Micro-pigmentation

Scalp micro-pigmentation is a non-surgical procedure that involves tattooing the scalp to create the appearance of hair follicles. The system uses specialized pigments and needles to create tiny dots that mimic the appearance of hair follicles. Scalp micro-pigmentation can make the appearance of a closely shaved head or add density to areas where hair is thinning.

Scalp micro-pigmentation is a low-risk procedure that can be completed in a single day. It can be a good option for individuals who do not want to undergo surgery or take medications. However, choosing a skilled and experienced practitioner is vital to ensure a natural-looking result.

Discussing these options with a qualified healthcare professional and making an informed decision based on individual circumstances is essential.

Medications, hair transplantation, and scalp micro-pigmentation are all effective treatments for hair loss, and the best approach will depend on the individual's needs and preferences.

In conclusion, several medical approaches to hair loss can help individuals restore their hair and improve their self-esteem.

Chapter 6

Staying Positive and Empowered: Tips and Strategies

Staying positive and empowered can be challenging when faced with a difficult situation like hair loss. Feeling self-conscious, vulnerable, and unsure of how to move forward is natural.

Still, it's important to remember that you are not alone in your journey and that there are many strategies you can use to stay positive and empowered.

Here are some tips and strategies for staying positive and empowered when living with hair loss:

1. **Practice gratitude**

Focusing on what you are grateful for can help shift your perspective and help you feel more positive and empowered. Each day, take a few minutes to reflect on the things you are grateful for, no matter how small they may seem.

2. **Set goals**

Setting goals can help you feel more in control of your situation and give you a sense of purpose and direction. Celebrate your accomplishments as you set short- and long-term goals.

3. Find ways to connect with others

Connecting with others going through similar experiences can be a powerful way to stay positive and empowered. Consider joining a support group or connecting with others online who are living with hair loss. Sharing your story and connecting with others can help you feel less alone and provide a sense of community and support.

4. Take care of yourself

Taking care of yourself is crucial for maintaining your emotional well-being. Caring for yourself might involve exercising, eating a healthy diet, or finding ways to relax and de-stress. It's essential to make time for self-care to cope with the challenges of living with hair loss.

5. **Seek support**

It can be helpful to seek support from friends, family, or a therapist as you work to cope with hair loss. Surrounding yourself with supportive people can help you feel less alone and provide a safe space to discuss your feelings and concerns.

6. **Find ways to connect with others**

Connecting with others going through similar experiences can be a powerful way to stay positive and empowered. Consider joining a support group or connecting with others online who are living with hair loss. Sharing your story and connecting with others can help you feel less alone and provide a sense of community and support. It can also be helpful to seek support from friends and family members who can provide emotional support and understanding.

7. *Take care of yourself*

Taking care of yourself is vital for maintaining your emotional well-being. Caring for yourself might involve exercising, eating a healthy diet, or finding ways to relax and de-stress. It's essential to make time for yourself as you strive to stay positive and empowered.

8. *Practice mindfulness*

Mindfulness is practicing paying attention to the present moment in a non-judgmental way. It can be a powerful tool for staying positive and empowered when living with hair loss. Consider incorporating mindfulness into your daily routine by setting aside a few minutes to focus on your breath, notice your surroundings, or engage in a calming activity like meditation or yoga.

9. Find ways to express yourself

Expressing yourself through art, writing, or other creative outlets can be a powerful way to cope with the emotional challenges of hair loss. Consider finding a creative outlet that resonates with you, and allow yourself the space to explore your feelings and emotions through art or writing.

10. Seek out positive role models

Surrounding yourself with positive role models can be a powerful way to stay positive and empowered. Look for people who have successfully navigated hair loss and can provide inspiration and guidance as you embrace your new identity.

11. Practice self-compassion

It's important to be kind to yourself as you navigate the challenges of living with hair loss. You can practice self-compassion by speaking to yourself in a kind and understanding or by reminding yourself that it's okay to feel a range of emotions as you adjust to your new identity.

Lifestyle Changes and Hair Loss

While hair loss is often associated with genetics or medical conditions, lifestyle factors can also play a role in hair health. In this section, we will explore how diet, exercise, and stress management can impact hair loss, and what changes individuals can make to promote hair health.

Diet

A balanced diet is essential for overall health, and it can also help promote healthy hair growth. Some nutrients that are particularly important for hair health include:

1. ***Protein:***

Hair is made of protein, so consuming adequate amounts of protein is essential for healthy hair growth. Protein sources include fish, lean meats, beans, eggs, and nuts.

2. *Iron:*

The iron in hair follicles helps carry oxygen. Iron plays an essential role in healthy hair growth. Good sources of iron include lean meats, seafood, beans, and dark leafy greens.

3. *Vitamins and minerals:*

Vitamins and minerals such as vitamins A, C, E, biotin, and zinc are also crucial for healthy hair growth. These nutrients can be found in various fruits, vegetables, and whole grains.

On the other hand, a diet that is high in processed foods, sugar, and unhealthy fats may contribute to hair loss. Consuming excessive amounts of alcohol or caffeine can also have a negative impact on hair health.

Exercise

Regular exercise is not only good for overall health but can also help promote healthy hair growth. Exercise improves blood flow and circulation, which can help deliver nutrients and oxygen to the hair follicles. Additionally, exercise can help reduce stress, a common cause of hair loss.

Stress Management

Stress can significantly contribute to hair loss, disrupting the normal hair growth cycle. Finding healthy ways to manage stress, such as exercise, meditation, or deep breathing exercises, can help promote healthy hair growth.

Other Lifestyle Factors

Other lifestyle factors that can impact hair health include:

1. *Hair care practices:*

Over washing, harsh chemicals and heat styling can all contribute to hair damage and hair loss. Gentle hair care practices (using mild shampoos, avoiding excessive heat, and avoiding harsh chemicals) can help promote hair health.

2. *Smoking:*

Smoking has been linked to hair loss, as it can damage the hair follicles and contribute to poor circulation.

3. **Sleep**:

Adequate sleep is essential for overall health and can help promote healthy hair growth. Lack of sleep can disrupt the normal hair growth cycle and contribute to hair loss.

In conclusion, lifestyle factors such as diet, exercise, and stress management can significantly impact hair health. Making healthy choices, such as consuming a balanced diet, engaging in regular exercise, and finding healthy ways to manage stress, can help promote healthy hair growth and reduce the risk of hair loss.

It is essential to discuss any concerns about hair loss with a qualified healthcare professional and make an informed decision about the best course of treatment.

Chapter 7

Living with Hair Loss: A Day in the Life

Living with hair loss can be a complex and emotionally challenging experience, and it's natural to feel self-conscious, vulnerable, and unsure of how to move forward. Throughout this chapter, you will be inspired by the strength and resilience of those who have faced hair loss and gain a greater understanding of this experience's impact on a person's life.

Here's a look at what a day in the life of someone living with hair loss might look like:

In the morning

1. Upon waking up, you might feel self-conscious about your appearance, mainly if you are used to wearing a wig or other form of head covering. You might take a few extra minutes to look in the mirror, reminding yourself that you are more than your appearance.

2. As you prepare for the day, you might take extra care in your grooming routine. This routine might involve using a gentle shampoo and conditioner, using a scalp massage oil or other nourishing treatment to stimulate blood flow and nourish the scalp, and styling

your hair in a way that feels comfortable and confident.

3. You might also take time to practice self-care in the morning, whether that means going for a walk, practicing yoga, or simply enjoying a cup of coffee in peace..

Throughout the day

1. As you go about your day, you might feel self-conscious or anxious about your appearance, especially if you are in a new or unfamiliar setting. You might find it helpful to remind yourself of your unique qualities and strengths and to focus on the things that make you special and unique.

2. You might also find it helpful to seek support from friends, family, or a therapist as you navigate the

challenges of living with hair loss. Surrounding yourself with supportive people can help you feel less alone and provide a safe space to discuss your feelings and concerns.

3. As you go about your daily activities, you might find it helpful to practice mindfulness, paying attention to the present moment in a non-judgmental way. This might involve focusing on your breath, noticing your surroundings, or engaging in calming activities like meditation or yoga.

In the evening

1. As you wind down for the day, you might find it helpful to set aside time for self-care, whether relaxing with a book, listening to music, or simply enjoying a warm bath.

2. You might also find it helpful to reflect on your day, focusing on the things you are grateful for and the positive aspects of your day. This can help you stay positive and empowered as you navigate

3. You might be dealing with negative comments or stares from others, which can be challenging. It can be helpful to remember that people's reactions are often driven by their insecurities and that you can choose how you respond to these situations.

4. You might try reminding yourself of your unique qualities and strengths or finding a supportive friend or loved one to talk to about your feelings.

What a Day in the Life of Someone Living with Hair Loss Looks Like

Here are some additional details on what a day in the life of someone living with hair loss might look like:

1. As you go about your daily activities, you might find it helpful to have strategies to manage your condition and maintain your emotional well-being. Managing your condition and maintaining your emotional well-being might involve finding a hairstyle that works for you, taking care of your scalp, seeking support, and practicing self-care.

2. You might also find it helpful to explore treatment options for hair loss, such as medications, hair transplant surgery, or scalp reduction surgery. It's essential to carefully consider these treatments'

pros and cons and work with a healthcare provider to determine the best course of action for your specific situation.

3. It can be helpful to have a supportive network of friends and loved ones who understand your hair loss experience and can provide emotional support and understanding. You might find it helpful to seek positive role models who have successfully navigated hair loss and can provide inspiration and guidance.

4. It's essential to remember that living with hair loss is a journey and that it's okay to have ups and downs along the way. It's important to be kind to yourself, to practice self-compassion, and to remember that it's okay to feel a range of emotions as you adjust to your new identity.

Living with hair loss can be a complex and emotionally challenging experience. Still, it's important to remember that you are not alone and that there are strategies you can use to stay positive and empowered.

By practicing gratitude, setting goals, seeking support, self-care, and seeking positive role models, you can navigate the challenges of living with hair loss and find confidence and empowerment in your new identity.

Personal Stories of Hair Loss

In this section, we will feature personal stories from individuals who have experienced hair loss. These stories will provide insight into the unique struggles and triumphs of those who have faced this challenging experience and offer tips and strategies for coping with hair loss.

Hair loss can profoundly impact a person's sense of self, confidence, and emotional well-being. While everyone's experience with hair loss is unique, hearing the stories of others who have gone through similar experiences can be both comforting and empowering.

The individuals we feature in this chapter come from diverse backgrounds, and their stories showcase various experiences with hair loss. Some of the topics covered in their stories include:

1. *Coping with the emotional impact of hair loss:*

Many of the individuals we feature in this chapter share the emotional toll that hair loss can take on a person's sense of self-worth, confidence, and emotional well-being. They offer insights into how they coped with these emotions and share tips for others who may be going through similar struggles.

2. *Finding support:*

Finding a support system can be a critical part of coping for many people with hair loss. Our featured individuals share their experiences finding support from loved ones, support groups, or online communities.

3. *Finding a sense of empowerment:*

While hair loss can be a challenging experience, many of the individuals we feature in this chapter also share stories of how they found a sense of empowerment in their journey. They offer tips for finding strength and resilience in the face of hair loss and showcase how this experience has helped them grow and evolve as individuals.

The personal stories shared in this section serve as a reminder that no one is alone in their struggles and that there is always hope for healing, growth, and self-empowerment.

Chapter 8

Finding Your Path Forward: Stories of Inspiration and Empowerment

Finding your path forward can be challenging, especially when faced with a difficult situation like hair loss. Feeling self-conscious, vulnerable, and unsure of how to move forward is natural.

Still, it's important to remember that you are not alone in your journey and that there are many inspiring and empowering stories of people who have navigated hair loss and found their path forward.

Inspirational Stories and Empowerment

Here are a few stories of inspiration and empowerment to consider:

Story #1

"My hair fell out as a result of chemotherapy, and that was a very emotional and difficult time for me. But I found strength and empowerment in the fact that I was fighting cancer and that my hair loss was a temporary side effect of treatment. I embraced my bald head and found ways to feel confident and comfortable in my skin. I also found support in a cancer support group and

my friends and family, who helped me navigate the challenges of living with hair loss. Today, I am cancer-free and have learned to embrace my new identity with confidence and grace." – **Makayla Persse.**

Story #2

"I experienced hair loss due to alopecia areata, an autoimmune disorder that causes hair loss. It was a difficult and emotional experience, and I struggled with self-consciousness and vulnerability. But I found strength and empowerment in the fact that I was not alone in my journey and that others were navigating similar challenges. I found support in a support group and my friends and family, and I learned to embrace my bald head confidently. I also found ways to express myself creatively through art and writing,

which helped me cope with the emotional challenges of living with hair loss. Today, I am confident and empowered in my new identity." – **Jasmine Clayton**

Story #3

"In my case, hair loss caused by male pattern baldness was emotionally and physically challenging. But I found strength and empowerment because I had control over my appearance, and treatment options were available to help me regrow my hair. I explored medications, hair transplant surgery, and scalp reduction surgery and ultimately decided on a treatment plan that worked best for me. I also found support from friends and family and learned to embrace my bald head confidently. Today, I am confident and empowered *in my new identity and am grateful for the journey that has brought me to where I am today." –* **Derek A. Delgadillo.**

By sharing these stories of inspiration and empowerment, we hope you will find encouragement and guidance as you navigate your journey with hair loss. Remember that you are not alone and that there are many strategies you can use to stay positive and empowered as you find your path forward.

Finding Support and Community

Hair loss can be an isolating experience, but finding support and community can help individuals feel less alone and more empowered in their journey. This section will provide resources for finding support and connecting with others who have experienced hair loss.

Online communities and forums can be valuable resources for individuals with hair loss. These groups allow people to connect with others who have gone through similar experiences and share tips, advice, and emotional support. Some popular online communities for individuals with hair loss include:

1. **The American Hair Loss Association forum:**

This forum offers a supportive community for individuals with hair loss as well as information on treatments, products, and resources.

2. **The Women's Hair Loss Project:**

This online community is specifically for women with hair loss, and provides a safe and supportive space for sharing stories and advice.

3. **The Bald Cafe:**

This forum is a supportive community for individuals who are bald or balding and includes discussions on various topics related to hair loss.

In addition to online communities, support groups can provide valuable in-person connections and support. These groups allow individuals to share their experiences with others face-to-face and can be a valuable source of emotional support.

Some organizations that offer support groups for individuals with hair loss include:

1. *Look Good, Feel Better:*

This organization offers free workshops, support groups for individuals with hair loss, and tips on skincare and makeup.

2. *The National Alopecia Areata Foundation (NAAF):*

This organization provides support groups for individuals with alopecia areata, as well as resources and information on treatments and research.

Finally, counseling can also be a valuable resource for individuals with hair loss. A licensed therapist can provide emotional support, coping strategies, and guidance on navigating hair loss's emotional and social challenges.

If you're interested in finding a therapist who specializes in hair loss, consider checking with a local support group or online community for recommendations.

In summary, finding support and community is integral to coping with hair loss. Whether you connect with others online, attend a support group, or seek counseling, it's essential to know that you're not alone and that resources are available to help you navigate this challenging experience.

Chapter 9

Embracing Your New Look

Hair loss can be a challenging experience, but it can also be an opportunity to embrace a new look and celebrate your unique style. This chapter will explore how to embrace and celebrate your new look after hair loss, including choosing flattering hairstyles, accessorizing, and dressing for your unique style.

Choosing a new hairstyle can be a fun and exciting part of embracing your new look. Many hairstyles can look great with short or no hair, such as a pixie cut, a buzz cut, or a shaved head. Consider wearing a wig or hairpiece, which can allow you to switch up your look and try different styles. When choosing a wig or hairpiece, consider the color, texture, and length, as well as the material and fit.

Accessories can also be fun to add personality and style to your new look. Scarves, headbands, and hats can be stylish and functional, keeping your head warm and protected from the sun. You may also want to experiment with bold jewelry, such as statement earrings or necklaces, to draw attention to your face and add a pop of color to your outfit.

When it comes to dressing for your new style, there are a few key things to keep in mind. First, consider your body type and choose clothing that flatters your shape. For example, if you have a round face, you may want to wear v-neck tops to elongate your neckline. If you have a more angular face, you should wear clothing with softer lines and curves to balance your features.

In addition, consider your style and choose clothing that makes you feel confident and comfortable. Considering your style may mean experimenting with new colors or styles or incorporating your favorite accessories or statement pieces into your new look.

Ultimately, embracing your new look after hair loss is about celebrating your unique style and personality. Whether you wear a wig, experiment with new hairstyles, or accessorize with bold jewelry and scarves, the most important thing is to feel confident and comfortable in your skin.

By embracing your new look and celebrating your individuality, you can turn a challenging experience into an opportunity for growth, self-expression, and self-love.

Advocacy and Empowerment

Hair loss can significantly impact an individual's self-esteem and confidence, but it's important to remember that you are not alone. Millions of people around the world experience hair loss, and together, we can work to raise awareness, promote understanding, and advocate for change.

This section will explore how individuals with hair loss can advocate for themselves and others, raise awareness about hair loss, and work to change societal attitudes and perceptions about baldness.

One way to advocate for yourself and others is by sharing your story. By speaking openly and honestly about your experiences with hair loss, you can help to break down the stigma and raise awareness about the impact that hair loss can have on an individual's mental health and well-being.

You can share your story with friends and family, on social media, or by participating in local or national hair loss awareness events.

Another way to advocate for change is by working to change societal attitudes and perceptions about baldness.

Changing societal attitudes and perceptions about baldness can involve challenging stereotypes, promoting diversity, and advocating for more representation in media and advertising. You can also work to change policies and laws that discriminate against individuals with hair loss, such as workplace dress codes or insurance coverage for wigs and hairpieces.

Advocacy can also involve supporting and empowering other individuals with hair loss. You can do this by participating in support groups, volunteering at local organizations that support individuals with hair loss, or simply offering a listening ear and a supportive word to those struggling with their own experiences.

Ultimately, advocacy and empowerment are about working together to create a world where all individuals feel accepted, valued, and supported, regardless of appearance. By advocating for yourself and others, you can help to break down barriers and promote understanding, paving the way for a more inclusive and compassionate society.

Conclusion

Going Bald with Grace is a comprehensive guide to navigating the challenges of living with hair loss and finding your own path forward with grace and confidence. Throughout the book, we have explored a range of strategies and techniques for staying positive and empowered as you embrace your new identity.

Here are a few key takeaways to consider as you reflect on the lessons of *Going Bald with Grace*:

- Practice gratitude
- Set goals
- Find ways to connect with others
- Take care of yourself
- Seek support

By incorporating these strategies into your daily routine, you can embrace your new identity with grace and confidence as you navigate the challenges of going bald. Remember that you are not alone in your journey and that there are many resources and support systems available to help you find your own path forward.

About the Author

Kayla S. Brigman is a health professional, author, speaker, and advocate for people with hair loss. After experiencing a loved one struggle with alopecia, she set out to learn more about the emotional and practical challenges of hair loss and to share her insights with others.

Kayla holds a degree in psychology and has worked as a counselor and coach, helping individuals navigate life transitions and build resilience. She has also contributed to various online publications and support communities, sharing her personal story and offering guidance on hair loss and self-care.

In "*Going Bald with Grace*," Kayla draws on her loved one's experiences and extensive research to offer practical strategies and heartfelt encouragement for individuals with hair loss. Her goal is to help readers find confidence, beauty, and power in their new look and to create a supportive and inclusive community that embraces diversity in all its forms.

Other Books by the Author

Below are other amazing book(s) by Kayla S. Brigman

BOOK TITLE	BOOK COVER	LINK TO READ
End The Snore Struggle	END THE SNORE STRUGGLE A Comprehensive Guide to Stopping Snoring and Improving Your Sleep Quality KAYLA S. BRIGMAN	Click Here to read for free on Kindle Unlimited
The Art of Being Fresh	KAYLA S. BRIGMAN THE ART OF BEING FRESH TIPS & TRICKS FOR BEATING BODY ODOR	Click Here to read for free on Kindle Unlimited

The Lean Body Blueprint	THE LEAN BODY BLUEPRINT — A STEP-BY-STEP GUIDE TO LOSING WEIGHT, BUILDING MUSCLE — KAYLA S. BRIGMAN	[Click Here to read for free on Kindle Unlimited](#)
Postpartum Body Rejuvenation For Women	POSTPARTUM BODY REJUVENATION FOR WOMEN — KAYLA S. BRIGMAN	[Click Here to read for free on Kindle Unlimited](#)
Kiss Bad Breath Goodbye	KISS BAD BREATH GOODBYE — THE ULTIMATE GUIDE TO ELIMINATING MOUTH ODOR — KAYLA S. BRIGMAN	[Click Here to read for free on Kindle Unlimited](#)

The Anti-Aging Blueprint	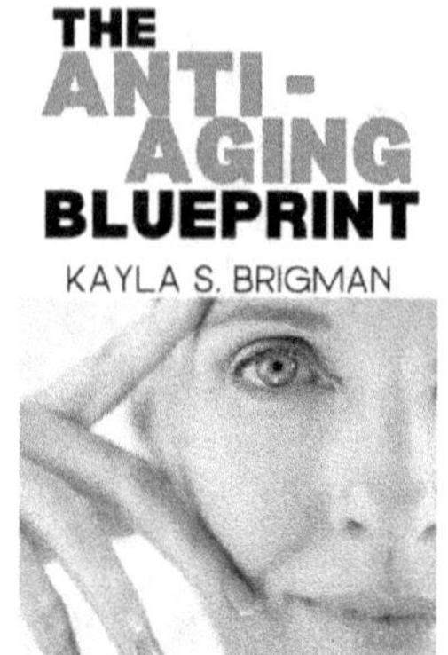	<u>Click Here to read for free on Kindle Unlimited</u>

THE END